I0837500

BECOMING YOU: A QUICK BEGINNER'S GUIDE TO MINIMALISM AND ZERO WASTE

AND A START TO LESS-ZERO WASTE EXISTENCE

By

DORION JARDIN

Copyright © 2018

Introduction

It is always a good time to think about creating an existence with zero waste. Know that it won't come easy and it won't happen overnight. And neither should it. In order to make any significant changes in your life and for it to have any lasting impact, one must implement and aim for a slow, thoughtful, and deliberate change.

Aim for achieving low to zero waste lifestyle. Some eco-friendly and zero waste tips are extremely easy, but it takes a little commitment to keep incorporating it in life. Remember that there isn't one correct way Sometimes there would more.

Knowing that there are a multitude of ways in which one can make a positive impact on the space surrounding us. These ways will range from options being the best, to better and worst. Making a conscious consumer is where you will be able to start making good choices.

So, start by making smaller, simpler choices today, and don't let a little effort prevent you from achieving a less wasteful existence.

TABLE OF CONTENTS

CHAPTER 1. ESTABLISH A WHY

Everyone who chooses to adopt a zero-waste lifestyle

almost always has a Why. Get specific about your

personal philosophy and your Why, so you are able to

turn it in your daily life as a powerful motivator.

Whether its concern for your environment, or your

need to get your spending under control, zero waste

is prudent for many reasons. Remember that this

lifestyle is healthier, and cheaper than you might think

at first.

Summary:

Establishing a Why will help you guide in your everyday life to achieve your goals of less waste lifestyle.

Chapter 2. Assess Your Waste

Start off by going through your trash. This will give you a good insight into what needs to be addressed, and the How will follow accordingly. Even if you find that there are some areas in which you feel you cannot possibly solve, by choosing to recycle or compost, you will be making a big difference than not doing anything at all.

Keep in mind the five R's: **Refuse, Reduce, Reuse, Recycle and Rot.**

All these R's must be applied together while accessing your waste, and in sequence.

Refuse so you will have less to Reduce, the more that is reduced, the less it leads to Reuse. Everything else then must get Recycled and composted so to Rot.

Do not accept something which would let to more demand. Apply the five R's not just to food waste but also before buying anything. This will help you save money, being easier on your wallet and health, as you will begin to swap out things to re-use from your waste.

Summary:

Adhere to the five R's before purchasing and afterwards. Incorporate this and make it your daily habit to encourage savings – saving money and saving the environment.

Chapter 3. Prioritise

Something as small as choosing to buy to-go coffee's or to order take out is wasteful. Packing a lunch, and taking a reusable mug from home, ensures better zero waste habits. Same goes for toiletries. Look at into buying from places that produce sustainably made products. Focus on to small areas of your life which produce waste, and it will not be overwhelming. Almost all areas of life has a sustainable way of procuring and/or disposing.

Summary:

When looking at the big picture of your waste, try and

divide it by area of needs. It will help bring things in

focus. Doing this will make you realise just how much

waste you are producing.

Chapter 4. Research How-To Recycle, Donate or Sell

But wait. Before you go throwing all your non-zero-waste items out, remember that it might not happen overnight. It just might take anywhere from a year or two to be fully zero waste compliant. And this is okay. Throwing away unused items is also quite wasteful. Find a way to reuse old items wherever you can. Use up as much as you can and think of better less to no waste alternatives for those items for next time.

Summary:

The goal here is to keep as many things out of landfills as possible. Keeping our oceans clean. Use these philosophies to ensure a cleaner environment not only for humans but for animals with whom we share this space with.

CHAPTER 5. REMEMBER THAT THIS IS ALL A PROCESS

Recycle whatever you can, compost whatever can be, and find a way to re-use or up-cycle whatever you can. If there is something which you do not want anymore, try to donate it or sell it. Do not let doing a little keep you away, as its all the little things that add up to make a massive impact.

Summary:

There are many people who take all sorts of materials

and turn them either into art or other usable items.

Look for these online.

CHAPTER 6. 50 THINGS TO START IMPLEMENTING RIGHT AWAY

Let make choices to make the world a little less wasteful, every day.

1. When out, do not get a plastic straw for your drink

2. Bring a reusable water bottle from home

3. Avoid using tissues by using handkerchiefs instead

4. Do not buy cheap items on promotion. They tend to be of bad quality and break easy

5. Donate unused items in good condition to support local markets

6. Think about purchasing something second-hand rather than brand new

7. Try swapping natural remedies before reaching for over-the-counter medications

8. Switch your plastic toothbrush for natural bamboo toothbrushes

9. Turn old bedsheets into handkerchiefs or rags to clean around the house

10. Wash clothes when they are dirty, instead of after each wear

11. Open a window to cool your home

12. Try to avoid using products with palm oil

13. Buy food items without or with minimal packaging

14. When feeling and instead of going for Retail Therapy, go for a walk or try yoga

15. Revive stale old bread instead of throwing it out

16. Use natural options as Dry Shampoo to prolong between washes

17. Try to streamline and buy items which have multiple uses

18. Try your hand at canning to preserve your food

19. Use a bar soap instead of liquid, it tends to have less packaging

20. Change your light bulbs to LED's

21. Be mindful when using technology, as E-waste is a growing segment of the municipal solid waste system

22. Bring reusable bag for produce and vegetables

23. Put on warm clothing before turning up the heat

24. Turn of the running water whenever you can during washing dishes or brushing teeth

25. Try not to buy anything on impulse

26. Try your hand at making your own, multi-purpose lotion

27. Check out your local farmer's markets as often as you can

28. Make facemasks from ingredients in your pantry

29. Get rid of pests, naturally

30. Plan your meals at home to avoid food waste

31. Unplug your electronics when they are not in use, even if you are still at home

32. Try to make your own tooth powder in order to avoid unrecyclable tooth paste tubes

33. Buy more locally made goods

34. Always try to opt for repairing something when it breaks

35. If looking for a specialty item, try to see if you are able to borrow it from a friend rather than purchasing it

36. Plant a small garden

37. Learn how to freeze your food so it doesn't go to waste, without the use of plastic

38. Make your own room and fabric fresheners for pennies

39. Start a backyard compost

40. Store your food properly to make it last longer

41. Find a local cobbler to repair shoes and handbags

42. Ask for no plastic or reused packaging materials where possible

43. Most sunscreen cause coral bleaching. Buy coral friendly sunscreen

44. Buy rechargeable batteries

45. Go paperless for all bills

46. Try to shrink what you have to recycle. Zero waste is about recycling less and not more.

47. Avoid getting receipts when out

48. Take public transport or carpool whenever possible

49. Join a community garden

50. Swap tea bags for loose-leaf tea

There are a lot of misconceptions attached to this lifestyle. People assume that this costs a lot more and takes too much time. Which is not the case, and is quite the opposite.

A less to zero waste lifestyle is a good choice for the environment, it is good for our health, and great for the planet.

No matter where you are in the world, you can refuse things which you don't need. Make sure to reduce the things which you actually need.

Find a system that works for you. Avoid going to such extremes where this is all consuming. Give yourself time, and learn to say no to unnecessary things.

www.ingramcontent.com/pod-product-compliance
Lightning Source LLC
Chambersburg PA
CBHW051145250726
48655CB00007B/3241